IN ALL
CIRCUMSTANCES

Lessons of Hope
in the Shadow of Illness

John Whaley with Mark Holt

To all those needing hope in the dark parts of their journey

&

To my mother who taught me the wisdom of hiding God's Word in my heart at a very young age.

ISBN 979-8-9874397-0-8

CONTENTS

Prologue 1

1 Something is Off 4

2 Breath 6

3 Trust - Know When to Fold 'em 12

4 Surrender 20

5 COVID Relief 24

6 A New Diagnosis 28

7 Quiet Time 32

8 COVID is the Best 38

9 Opportunity 42

10 Chemo and Red 46

11 On Assignment 52

12 From the Mind of God 58

13 A Possibility of Hope 60

14 Little Bunny and the Big Bad Giant 68

15 God's Kindness 72

16 Mantel Cell Lymphoma is Gone 76

17 The Boogeyman Defeated Again 80

18 Oh, by the Way, You Have Brain Cancer ... 86

19 Praying for Healing 90

20 Fear and Discouragement 96

21 A Devastating Diagnosis 100

22 Is This God's Fault? 106

23 Difficult Decisions 108

24 Continuing the Fight 112

25 Is There Still Hope for Healing? 116

26 Looking to My Future 120

I'm Dying

Hi, my name is John and I'm dying.

I don't mean to be morbid, but that's the truth of it. I don't know exactly when or from what. I'm in a battle with cancer right now. COVID and I already had a long tussle and I managed to stagger away from that one. (I'll tell you the whole story.) But, it is a fact that I will die from something - someday.

There's another ugly truth. We all have that same monkey on our back. We're all dying. I know. I sell life insurance. In the business, we call it 'end of plan.' Most people don't like to deal with it and try not to think about it until they're in a position like mine. Because of my illnesses I've been forced to stare my own mortality in the face.

But I want to let you in on a little secret. I'm having the time of my life. As I was fighting COVID and then through the first stages of my cancer treatment, I felt like I was stumbling through a dark foggy woods, bouncing off trees, trying to find my way. Now, it seems like I've stepped out into an open meadow with bright sunshine and brilliant colors. Everything is vivid and rich. I wouldn't trade where I am in life.

Do I wish that I didn't have cancer? Of course! But it's often from dark places and deep trials that we come to know God better. Trials magnify the greatness of God. In this last year of fighting for my life, I have treasured his company and come to love him more than ever.

So why write a book like this? After all, there is nothing particularly unique about my story. A lot of people are diagnosed with a terminal illness. Many are treated and recover. Many do not. But as I've talked to people about God's hand in my journey, many have asked me to write it down. They seem to be encouraged by someone in the middle of the fight whose faith transcends circumstances. Life beats us down and we all need a friendly and inspiring word to help us press on. If I can be an encourager to someone in the middle of their own battle, it would make it all worthwhile.

I also want to finish my life well (whenever that is). You may be young or old, perfectly healthy or facing a terminal disease, but if you allow yourself to think about it, I'm sure you want your life to count. You want to finish well too. That means living well in whatever stage of life you are at. In the following pages, I hope to pass along some important lessons that are helping me draw closer to God, live a life of gratitude and purpose, and stay on assignment – In All Circumstances.

John Whaley

3   SOMETHING IS OFF

Something is Off

I woke up Monday morning and something felt off. It was nothing dramatic but I felt different, kind of blah. I told my wife, Sharon, that I was only 70% of what I normally am, and since I don't usually give her a score first thing in the morning it made me pay attention.

I continued to feel that way for the next couple days. I had some client meetings and went to choir practice at church Wednesday night. I didn't bother taking a COVID test since there was disagreement about their accuracy at the time. Then Thursday and Friday I really started to feel bad, but I still wanted to get some things done, including signing papers on our new house in Florida.

The next week got worse. I continued downhill fast and my breathing became labored. I finally took a COVID home test from the drugstore and it revealed the dreaded news that both Sharon and I had COVID. She felt miserable but, thankfully, wasn't struggling to breathe. I was clearly on a downward trend but both the government and the health officials were telling people to stay home and ride it out.

After a couple more days I couldn't take it any longer. I couldn't breathe. I didn't even want to get out of bed anymore. It was getting dangerous. On Thanksgiving Day around 6:30 in the evening, I told Sharon I needed to go to the ER.

The waiting room was filled with people all wearing masks and a look of desperation on their faces. The hospital was overrun with COVID patients. Staff wearing double gowns and gloves, face shields and masks circulated through the crowd, making sure the most serious patients got help immediately. They must have seen something in my condition because I was whisked away into a triage room and tested for COVID. They put an oxygen mask over my mouth and nose and, for the first time in days, I felt some relief.

At 1:30 in the morning they moved me up to room 302. It wasn't intensive care, but it was just one step below that. Maybe the reality of it hadn't hit yet, but I wasn't particularly frightened. The oxygen helped me breathe so I felt okay for the time being. Whatever happened, would happen, whether I worried about it or not.

What I didn't know was that I wouldn't leave room 302 until December 19th – 25 days later.

Breath

I couldn't get enough oxygen on my own anymore. Even with the cannula in my nose delivering a steady stream, I struggled to breathe. They started me off with 40-50ml of oxygen, but quickly had to increase the volume to keep me alive. I was heading toward the threshold of 70-80ml per minute where intubation was the inevitable next step. I was racing down a path I definitely didn't want to be on.

The Respiratory Therapy Department was involved from my first day. They had me use a device called a spirometer which was supposed to help expand my lungs. It was extremely uncomfortable and difficult to use. I exhaled through my nose and then slowly inhaled through a tube in my mouth. A piston in the spirometer would rise with each breath. I was supposed to get it as high in the tube as possible, but I had to be careful not to breathe too fast or too slow. An indicator to the right of the tube traveled up or down between two arrows with each breath. If it went above the top arrow, I was breathing too fast. If it fell below the bottom, I was breathing too slowly.

Then they wanted me to lay on my stomach, again to expand my lungs, but that made it even more difficult to breathe. By the third or fourth night, they put one of those fighter pilot masks over my nose and mouth to force more oxygen into my system. That made sleep next to impossible. Although the increased oxygen was a relief, the mask was loud and uncomfortable. The flow of life-giving oxygen roared in my ears and kept me awake. That's when I realized for the first time that I was speeding toward the brink of life and death and peeking over the edge into the abyss. I wondered what was happening to me.

It was during those long nights that I started to think about breath. After all, that's all my life was focused on at the moment. The sensor on my finger monitored how much oxygen was in my system. If something unplugged or if my level dropped below ninety percent, alarms sounded, equipment started beeping, and I was startled back to consciousness from whatever shallow sleep I was in. The nurses would rush in and tell me to breathe deeply through my nose to get the level back up and silence the alarms.

My lungs just weren't taking in the oxygen like they should. If I moved or rolled over in bed, it forced my heart to pump faster, which used more oxygen. My level would drop, the sensor would sound the alarm, and the nurses rushed in again urging me to breathe. It was a vicious cycle.

I became aware that something that had been automatic and involuntary all my life was now the sole focus of my attention. I was close to desperation. I was also keenly aware that I was alone. So, I talked to God about it. My prayer was pretty simple. *God, I can't breathe. If the breathing stops, there's nothing I can do about it. I am totally in your hands. This night is going to be long and any breath I get is from you. I can't do this.*

I never heard the audible voice of God that night, and I wasn't really looking for an answer. I just wanted to tell him what was on my plate and that whatever happened was okay with me. I did, however, ask him to help me breathe and help me get through it. I didn't need a big announcement from him. I just needed help breathing.

I slept fitfully for a little while and then woke up around 2:00am thinking more about breath. What did the Bible have to say about breath?

I thought about Adam. When God created him, he breathed life into him.

I thought of Ezekiel in the valley of dry bones. The Spirit of God breathed life into them.

Then I thought of Jesus. After his resurrection, he breathed on his followers, and they received the Holy Spirit.

But I thought most about Adam. I personally believe in the creation account in Genesis, so when the Bible says Adam was created out of the dust of the earth, I believe it's true. Now, it was 2:00 in the morning and I had nowhere else to go so I let my mind wander. What did that look like? I don't know the details, of course, but I believe that God made a form of man out of the dust and then he breathed life into it. Adam was "breathed" into life. And if he was created out of dirt, did he cough up a little dust after God breathed life into him?

When did Adam become aware of himself? The rest of us are born as babies and we don't become self-aware until much later. Some people never do. When did it happen for him? What was his first cognitive thought? Did he think, "Who am I?" first or about his surroundings first? Did he see and understand God? I can picture Adam waking up and saying, "Who am I?" Then seeing God and asking, "Who are you?" Then looking around at the garden and asking, "What am I doing here?"

It struck me that those are the questions everybody has to answer in life.

Who am I?

Who is God?

What am I doing here? What's my purpose?

Before I drifted off to a shallow sleep, I repeated my prayer, *God, I am totally in your hands. Any breath I get is from you. I need your help. I can't do this.*

◆

Sometimes in the middle of a crisis, all you can do is breathe and allow God to work. Like Adam, God gives you breath to give you life and to fill you with life.

Reflect on:

Who am I?

Who is God?

What is my purpose?

11 TRUST - KNOW WHEN TO FOLD 'EM

Trust - "Know When to Fold 'em"

My body was reaching tipping points I wasn't familiar with. Things were getting serious very quickly. I asked the doctor, "What's next if this stuff isn't working?"

He looked at me intently. "Intubation." Then we discussed what that meant.

"I don't think I want that."

"Okay," he said. "We can put that on your wrist. Do not intubate. But then your body is going to do whatever it's going to do."

"My next stop is better than this one anyway, so I guess I'm okay with that."

I probably wasn't aware of the magnitude of what I was saying in the heat of battle, but that's how I felt.

The doctor stared at me again. "We're not quite there yet."

We talked for a while longer. I wasn't overly emotional. I was just being logical because all I really wanted was the facts. Was I giving up? Not necessarily, but I wanted that as an option. Unfortunately, when my family found out about my conversation, they got really concerned. On my CaringBridge site, which provided friends and family with updates on my condition, my son, David, titled the entry for that day, "Know when to hold 'em. Know when to fold 'em," after the Kenny Rogers' song.

When I was a young boy my mother encouraged me to memorize a verse that has now become my life verse. Proverbs 3:5,6 (NKJV), "Trust in the Lord with all your heart and lean not on your own understanding; in all your ways acknowledge Him and He shall direct your paths." I clung to that truth as I weighed my medical choices: pursue any and all treatment options to stay alive or to release my grasp on this earth and let God take me home in his time. I was open to either one.

Through most of my life, however, I've been more than happy to give God a list of suggestions on how he should help me. After all, I believed, God gave me certain abilities. It only made sense that I should figure out what I can do myself and then trust God for the things I have no control over. The problem is, as I get older I realize I don't have control over any of it – especially when I'm in the hospital struggling to breathe. The only thing I can control is my attitude.

I first started to learn the lesson of trust during the housing crisis of 2008. We had our own financial catastrophe and I couldn't see any way out of it. We bought a beautiful condo in Minnesota in 2004 with an interest-only loan, knowing that we could always refinance to a traditional mortgage. In 2006, at the very peak of the market, we also borrowed a lot of money to buy a house in Florida. What we didn't know at the time was that the house was finished with toxic Chinese drywall.

Two years later the bottom fell out of the housing market and suddenly our Florida house was worth half of what we paid for it. Because of the Chinese drywall that destroyed everything it touched and made the house unsafe to live in, the value dropped to only fifteen percent of what we paid. Then, at the same time, the note on our Minnesota condo came due and there was no financing to be found. Banks stopped funding mortgages. Our monthly payments swelled to over $10,000.

We were swimming in an ocean of debt and I felt like I was being sucked down the drain after someone pulled the plug.

One friend offered to rescue me by cosigning a loan, but when Sharon and I prayed about it, we decided it was unwise for him to hitch his wagon to my falling star. No need to drag someone else down with me.

Then we met for three and a half hours with a financial advisor. His idea was to make me look really poor on my balance sheets, like I didn't have any assets, even though I did. From there we would go into bankruptcy, foreclosure, or whatever would be necessary to get out from under our financial burdens. Needless to say, we didn't have to pray about that plan for very long.

It was the Friday night of Memorial Weekend 2009 that we learned our house was built with toxic drywall. I was sound asleep until I woke in a panic at 2:00am, feeling like someone had put the defibrillator pads on my chest to kickstart my heart. I gasped as my eyes flew open to a dark room. I stared up toward the ceiling. *This is bad!. What am I going to do?* Then a calmer reminder came into focus. *Oh, yeah, I need to trust God. But what does that mean? We hear about it all the time, but what does it really mean? How do I do that?* My breathing started to slow and come back under control.

My first thought was to *Be Thankful.* I Thessalonians 5:18 (NIV) says"...give thanks in all circumstances; for this is God's will for you in Christ Jesus." It didn't say, "in most things." It wasn't just meant for when I feel good. It said in all circumstances. It was counter-intuitive but a lot of things in faith appear that way. I wanted to know and do the will of God and here was the first step spelled out for me. Give thanks in all circumstances, even the ones caused by our own bad decisions.

I continued to think of scripture that applied to my situation. 1 Peter 5:7 (NIV) tells us to, "Cast all your anxiety on Him because He cares for you." In order to do that, I have to trust him. I have to be totally reliant on him. I love the image of throwing all my worries on God, and my loving Abba Father will help take care of them.

"Come to Me, all you who are weary and burdened, and I will give you rest. Take My yoke upon you and learn from me, for I am gentle and humble in heart, and you will find rest for your souls. For My yoke is easy and My burden is light." Matthew 11:28-30 (NIV)

My worry, my anxiety…my trust, are spiritual things. I have to turn them over to God, first of all, because he cares, and second, because he promises to help.

We all need an arsenal of verses like this to go to when we get stuck. Satan works most effectively when we are discouraged or afraid. Memorized Bible verses are the climbing pegs I hold onto to help pull me out of the muck and mire of emotional despair and lift my thoughts up where they belong. I keep adding to my arsenal as time goes on.

In those agonizing days and weeks of our financial crisis I learned to trust God. There are consequences to our decisions, but God even helps with some of those outcomes because of his grace and mercy. Nothing God does is ever bad. Nothing!

We soldiered on, trusting God with the process and timing. We tapped all of our retirement accounts to continue making payments until, finally, we sold the condo. The toxic home in Florida took a couple more years to resolve, but eventually that too was fully repaired by the builder and eventually sold.

God rescued us and we learned to trust him in the process.

Those lessons, and the reassurance of God's deliverance from previous trials, calmed my mind on that Thanksgiving Day when I went into the hospital and had nothing left except trust. I didn't have strength. I didn't have any answers. I was quickly running out of breath. I prayed, *Lord, I'm here. If I float, it's because of you. If I sink, it's because of you. I'm totally dependent on you because I can't do anything for myself.*

After my discussion with the doctor about my options, I asked for a visit from the palliative care staff. They're the people who keep you comfortable when you're dying. At the time, most of those visits were virtual because of COVID, but a very nice woman went through the bother of gowning and masking up and talking with me in person for about forty-five minutes.

"What happens if I stop doing all this stuff? Do you just keep me comfortable?

She said, "It's not quite that simple. Hospice is for people who are going to live six months or less. We'd have to make a special request for that."

As she was describing all the steps necessary to get me into hospice, it sounded like more work to start dying than to just do what they were already asking me to do. So I relented. "Okay, okay. Never mind. I'll do what I need to do."

The next morning the doctor came in to check on me. "How do you feel? Are you in pain? How are your bowel movements? (For some reason they were very interested in my bowel movements.)

"You know, I feel pretty good. I had a really good bowel movement this morning. I also talked to the palliative care people yesterday and I got rid of all that crap too. I'm good to go. I'm on board with anything we need to do."

That was the first time I'd seen him smile in days.

On my CaringBridge page, my son concluded, "As far as hold 'em or fold 'em? We're going to hold 'em."

◆

Make it a regular practice to give God thanks, not *for* all circumstances, but *in* all circumstances. Start a list of the things you are thankful for.

Satan is most effective when you are afraid or discouraged. He is actively working to find ways to undermine your faith and replace it with fear and discouragement.

When you are empty, with nothing left, you can fully lean on God for help. He will direct your path. (Prov. 3:5,6)

Surrender

As I lay in my hospital bed with oxygen being forced into my lungs, hooked up to an array of equipment monitoring my bodily functions, surrender took on a very special meaning. Under normal circumstances, we have time to think and process, weigh our options and then, hopefully, decide to surrender to God and his will. In the hospital, there was nothing I could do on my own. My strength was already stripped away. My body couldn't function on its own. I wasn't waving a white flag. I had no flag. I was already surrendered. My life verse, Proverbs 3:5,6 (NKJV) starts with, "Trust in the Lord with all your heart, and lean not on your own understanding." Well, I had no understanding. I was wide-eyed dependent on God for my next breath.

I suppose I could have turned and shaken my fist at God. I could have been defiant and demanded to know why he would do this to me. Even in my condition, it was still a choice. *God*, I prayed, *I give up. I give in. You win. I lose. I am totally surrendered to you.*

There is nothing else I can do.

My wife had been talking to a friend of ours who had survived her own battle with COVID. She wanted to encourage me and she didn't mince words. "John, you can do this. You have to do this! But you have to be intentional about doing what they say. You can get out of the hospital and get your life back." Then she gave me three scripture verses. Psalm 118:17 (NKJV) "I shall not die but live, and declare the works of the Lord." Exodus 23:25,26 (NKJV) "So you shall serve the Lord your God, and He will bless your bread and your water. And I will take sickness away from the midst of you. No one shall suffer miscarriage or be barren in your land; I will fulfill the number of your days." 1 Peter 2:24 (NKJV) "...who Himself bore our sins in His own body on the tree, that we, having died to sins, might live for righteousness–by whose stripes you were healed." (I prefer to say, *by whose stripes I am healed.*) God used her in that conversation to convince me that I could do this. I had to do it!

In the end, surrender was easy for me because I didn't have anything to fight with. I didn't even have anything to give up. It was already gone. I clung to the second part of those verses from Proverbs, "In all your ways acknowledge Him, and He shall direct your paths." That's the only hope I had.

But it required action on my part. I still struggled to breathe, lying on my stomach, forcing air into my lungs to keep the alarms from sounding, watching the piston in the spirometer rise and fall, expanding my lungs and praying that God would give me my next breath.

In those early days in the hospital they also took a chest x-ray to see what COVID was doing to my lungs. It was common for the disease to fill the lungs with fluid or to actually crystalize lung tissue. What they found instead was a one-inch growth in my upper-right lung.

They called in a pulmonologist. He examined my x-ray on the light box, leaning his head back to look through his bifocals, and frowning deeply. He pointed to the white spot. "There's this one-inch thing. I'm pretty sure you came in with it, but I don't know what it is. It could be one of eight things." He went through the whole list but, again, said he didn't know for sure what it was. "We'll treat it like a bacterial or fungal infection and see if that clears it up."

They gave me some powerful horse pills and steroids, but it didn't change a thing. The mass stayed right where it was. When my COVID emergency was over, the doctors would have to take a closer look.

In the meantime, I had to keep breathing.

◆

When it seems that your life is falling apart, you can still experience God's loving care.

There will be times of hardship, loss and waiting, but God can use your situation to accomplish his purpose in your life.

COVID Relief

It was mid-December and I had become pretty comfortable in room 302. My breathing was starting to come easier and they were able to slowly cut back on my oxygen. I was close to being able to breathe on my own, but the threshold for oxygen assistance before they would even start to consider releasing me was 20%. I finally clawed my way below that line on December 18th. After final examinations and approvals from my doctors, I was released the next day, 25 days after I first walked in.

When I got home I looked in the mirror. My Olympic athlete body was gone. My muscles were atrophied and seemed to hang from my frame. It exhausted me to stand there even with the cannula in my nose supplying a steady stream of oxygen. My energy level hovered at a dismal 2 out of 10, but I had a goal. We had a trip to Florida planned for the 15th of January to visit the house we closed on right before I went into the hospital. In my current condition, there was no way I'd be able to make the trip. I couldn't walk 100 steps without stopping, let alone walk through an airport, down the causeway and onto the plane. It just wouldn't be possible. I had work to do.

The Mall of America is located in a suburb of Minneapolis about 15 minutes from my house. One lap around the ground floor of the huge complex is just over a mile. That mile became the Everest I needed to summit. When I first attempted it, we had to stop five times to rest as I was completely exhausted and out of breath. But we walked every day and slowly my body got stronger and my breathing came easier.

It looked like I was going to survive COVID, but now my doctors turned their attention to the new threat. There was still that little one-inch mass in my right lung. Before the end of the year I had a CT scan and then on January 13th, they did a bronchoscopy and a biopsy of some of the lymph nodes around my lung. It would be a couple of weeks before we got any results and a clearer picture of what we were dealing with.

In the meantime, Sharon and I kept walking. In the midst of a bitter Minnesota winter, the Mall of America was our daily climb. The summit of completing a one-mile lap was finally conquered, and a week later I walked two full laps without stopping at all.

We took our trip to Florida.

◆

Oftentimes, our faith will be tested after God saves our lives and delivers us from the initial trial. We return to "normal" life, but with lingering challenges. It becomes a new phase in our faith journey.

Have you been disappointed that God has delivered you but not completely restored you?

What is God asking you to do? What next step do you need to partner with God on in your life?

A New Diagnosis

Sharon and I sat in the oncologist's office at Fairview Hospital waiting for the results of the tests and scans of my lungs. We squeezed each other's hand a little tighter as the doctor entered and closed the door behind her. There was no smile on her face.

"Here's what I think you have," she said. "It's mantel cell lymphoma, which is an aggressive type. Yours is stage four." Sharon and I looked at each other and braced ourselves. "It's not curable, but it is treatable."

"And if I don't do anything?" I asked. "How long do I have?"

"Somewhere in the range of 18 months."

"And if I do treat it?"

"We don't know for sure, but I'd estimate 3-5 years."

The doctor explained that mantel cell lymphoma is a type of non-Hodgkin's lymphoma that affects the white blood cells in lymph nodes. The cancer cells tend to multiply quickly and spread through the lymph system to other parts of the body. That's why my case was already considered stage four.

The weight of the diagnosis settled heavily on us. It was a bleak outlook and the doctor didn't give us much hope to hang on to. I could tell Sharon was crushed with the news. In just a few words, life for us was changed forever. After surviving my battle with COVID, I now faced a new death sentence from an incurable cancer.

The next day, I decided to drive up to our cabin thinking it would be a good place to process everything and spend time praying. God and I both enjoy our times together in the woods and on the water. The phone rang as I drove. It was a good friend from Little Falls, Minnesota and, of course, he asked me how I was feeling.

"I feel fine," I said. "I'm not feeling any of the effects of what's apparently happening in my body."

"I guess that's good," he said.

We talked for a couple of minutes, and I explained more of what the doctor told us. Then I paused for a second. "If it's that dire of a prognosis, I really don't need to go through all those gyrations and all that pain just to add six months to my life."

My friend didn't hesitate a second to hit me over the head with a proverbial 2x4. "John, this is not about you."

"What do you mean? Of course it's about me. I'm a Baby Boomer."

He wasn't distracted by my attempt at humor. "No, it's not about you. You have a sphere of influence. You have people watching you. Your job is to take the treatment, do your part, and trust God for the rest. The results are up to God. You don't get to pick the time. You just have to keep on trucking."

I drove in silence for a moment allowing his reproof to sink in. I wasn't necessarily set on doing nothing, but my friend's words were enough to jar me to a different way of thinking. "You're right," I said. "I'm not going to do that. Why am I sitting here thinking about philosophical things and giving up? We'll do what we can do."

"That's more like it," he said.

We met for lunch at a restaurant close to the cabin the following day, talking for at least another hour before it was time to leave. Our cars were parked on opposite sides of the lot so we had to walk in different directions once we exited the door. I could tell that he was reluctant to part ways. I'm sure he was having a hard time with a diagnosis that could potentially remove me from his life. He started to walk to his car and then stopped and turned in the middle of the parking lot. "You don't get to walk away from me," he pointed his finger. "You don't get to not talk to me. I get to talk to you."

I nodded and smiled, trying to assure him.

The next day I called Mayo to get a second opinion.

With God's help, I was able to get an appointment at Mayo for my first consultation on February 1st. The next day they performed an MRI, bone marrow biopsy and a colonoscopy. It was a full day of tests. Two weeks later the results came back and the doctor confirmed the initial diagnosis. I had stage four mantel cell lymphoma. One week later, on February 22nd, I was scheduled for my first chemo treatment.

My COVID journey may have been over, but my cancer journey was just beginning.

---◆---

Sometimes the bad news just keeps coming and you may be tempted to give up.

The lessons from your initial trial can help you face continued challenges.

It's not about you; it's about the work God still has for you.

God puts people in our lives to challenge us, support us and, sometimes, correct us. Who are those people in your life and are you open to their council?

Quiet Time

God gave me a wonderful gift at the start of my battle with cancer. It came in my morning quiet time on the day I was scheduled to have my first PET scan. I've made it a practice most of my life to spend time with God in his Word every day. Most mornings I have a set method of study, but on that morning as I was thinking about my situation, scripture came to mind and I followed where it led me.

I started by writing down the issues I was concerned about. First, I had a possible lymphoma for which I was having a PET scan later that day. The second issue looming in my mind was our upcoming move to Florida. There were huge obstacles and logistics to overcome and organize in a short period of time. Together, the issues kept my mind busy with the big "what ifs."

Hebrews 13:5b (NIV) came to mind. "Never will I leave you; never will I forsake you." So I concluded with confidence that the Lord is my helper.

I wrote down **Principal #1 - God is with me.**

Another set of verses popped into my memory. Matthew 7:7-11 (NIV) "Ask and it will be given to you; seek and you will find; knock and the door will be opened to you. For everyone who asks receives; the one who seeks finds; and to the one who knocks, the door will be opened.

Which of you, if your son asks for bread, will give him a stone? Or if he asks for a fish, will give him a snake? If you, then, though you are evil, know how to give good gifts to your children, how much more will your Father in heaven give good gifts to those who ask Him!"

I jotted down **Principal #2 – God tells us to ask, seek and knock. He has good gifts to give us.**

Psalm 18:30 (NIV) was a great reassurance of God's trustworthiness. "As for God, His way is perfect."

Then he seemed to lead me to a scripture that has always fascinated me and one I've never heard anyone talk about. 2 Kings 13:14 (NIV) says, "Now Elisha was suffering from the illness from which he died." If you remember, Elisha was Elijah's protégé who had asked for a double portion of what his master had in life. When Elijah was taken up to God and his mantle was placed on Elisha's shoulders, he received his request. It was almost as if Elisha had a double portion of the relationship with God that Elijah had.

What amazed and puzzled me about the story was that if a person had that kind of connection with God, why would they be suffering from a terminal illness? Wouldn't it make sense that God would heal them or prevent them from getting a disease in the first place?

Then I noticed another important point. Even as Elisha was suffering from a terminal condition, he was doing the work he was assigned to do. He was God's prophet, engaged in important matters with the king of Israel. He wasn't at home complaining about how unfair his circumstances were. He was busy doing the Lord's work until the day he died.

Principal #3 - There are some things that God does not keep from us – like illness. Even the apostle Paul had a thorn in the flesh. Scripture says, "It is appointed unto man once to die." Lazarus, who had been raised once from the dead, was not even immune. Apparently, it was appointed unto Lazarus to die twice.

So what was I supposed to learn from my circumstances? What was God trying to teach me on that morning? He brought me back again to Proverbs 3:5,6 (NKJV) "Trust in the Lord with all your heart, and lean not on your own understanding; in all your ways acknowledge Him, and He shall direct your paths."

Lesson #1 Trust Me

James 1:2,3 (NIV) also came to mind. "Consider it pure joy,

my brothers and sisters, whenever you face trials of many kinds, because you know that the testing of your faith produces perseverance." The King James version uses "patience" in place of "perseverance."

Lesson #2 Be patient and persevere

I had listened to a message from Chuck Swindoll a couple of weeks earlier that also applied to my situation. He spoke on Psalm 139, stating that God had prearranged my course, my race. Every day of my life had been planned by God before I was born. Psalm 139:16 (NIV) states, "…all the days ordained for me were written in Your book before one of them came to be." This is not some random walk through the wilderness for me. God has planned my days. He knew about my cancer long before my diagnosis.

Swindoll also pointed out that preparing for the race was my responsibility. I needed to have scripture in my memory to face the trials ahead.

I also needed to stay focused on Jesus, not get distracted, and whenever I would get discouraged (which was bound to happen), think of what Jesus endured. Quitting wouldn't make it any easier. Finish the race. Finish it well. And don't give up!

I wrote all those points down and then made this conclusion – **The only thing I have control over is my attitude.**

My attitude is based on the conviction that:

God's way is perfect – Psalm 18:30

His word is flawless – Psalm 18:30

God is good – Psalm 100:5

God's grace is sufficient – 2 Corinthians 12:9

God's mercy is everlasting – Psalm 100:5

God is always with me – Deut. 31:6 & Isaiah 41:10

God promises to help me – Hebrews 13:6 & Psalm 18:6

My times are in his hands – Psalm 31:15

Our God is in the heavens and does whatever he pleases – Psalm 115:3

God has a plan for me – Jeremiah 29:11

I finished my quiet time with Psalm 20:7 (NIV), "Some trust in chariots and some in horses, but we trust in the name of the Lord our God." And Zechariah 4:6b (NIV), "Not by might nor by power, but by my Spirit, says the Lord Almighty."

I understood my quiet time that morning as God speaking directly to me, preparing me for what lay ahead. It set the tone for my attitude in the months to follow. I now realize how much I needed those verses.

———————————————◆———————————————

Write down the issues you are concerned about and then reflect on the truths he has revealed:

- God is with you. He will never leave you or forsake you. He is your helper.
- God wants us to ask, seek and knock. He has good gifts for us.
- There are some things that God may not keep from us - like illness.
- Trust God.
- Be patient and persevere.
- The only thing you have control over is your attitude.

COVID is the Best

"COVID is the best thing that ever happened to me."

"What are you talking about?"

"Well, if I hadn't had COVID and been in the hospital, they wouldn't have found out I have cancer."

"And that's a good thing?" The man shook his head, wondering what kind of weirdo he was talking to.

I was on my first bike outing after my initial chemo treatment in late February of 2022. I wanted to do what the old guys do around our neighborhood here in Fort Myers, Florida, which is ride my bike about five miles up to the McDonalds, eat a cinnamon roll, and then ride back home.

I have two bicycles. One is a road bike which, when I was healthy and in shape, I could get up to a speedy 17 miles an hour. But I haven't done that for at least a year so the tires are flat on that one.

My second bike is an old balloon-tire Schwinn cruiser. I call it my Buick LeSabre of bicycles. It's big and cushy. It creaks and groans. It's built for comfort, not speed. But I can get somewhere if I give myself enough time, and that's exactly what I was doing that morning. After enjoying my cinnamon roll, I was on my way back home, riding on a long straight stretch of sidewalk that parallels the highway. It was a typical Fort Myers morning. The rising sun pulled temperatures into the mid-seventies and spotty clouds gave me brief islands of shade along my path. I was probably cruising at six or seven miles an hour, just enjoying the morning sunshine, when a guy went huffing and puffing by me at least twice my speed on a mountain bike. He wheezed out a "good morning," as he flew by on my left.

I yelled back, "It's a great morning!"

He slammed on his brakes, even though he was already well past me by that point, and let me catch up to him. I guess my exuberance about the day made him curious.

We got to chatting with the standard questions. Where are you from? What are you doing? He mentioned that he had some kind of heart issue and it was one of the reasons he was out biking. That's when I noticed his compression socks. "How about you?" He asked.

"Well, I used to do a lot more biking but I've been kind of sidetracked with COVID."

"Oh?"

Yeah, I was in the hospital for 25 days."

"Oh, no."

"I lost my Olympic-athlete body."

"Oh, no," he said again, even though I'm sure he had his doubts.

"But you know what? It was the best thing that ever happened to me."

"Huh?" His faced scrunched up, but I could tell he was curious.

"Yeah, if I hadn't had COVID and been in the hospital, they never would have found out I have cancer."

"That's a good thing?"

"Yeah, because if I hadn't found that out, the cancer would have kept on growing until it was too late. Now, I know it's treatable. I could live a long time with it. I'm grateful for COVID."

I could tell he was having a hard time processing my positive attitude after such a devastating diagnosis. We talked more about it and I did my best to explain what was going on in my body. "Either way," I said, "it's a win/win for me. If the cancer gets stalled, that's great. But if it doesn't…" I shrugged my shoulders. "I'm going to heaven anyhow. And that's much better. It's a win/win."

The man listened as we pedaled together for a couple more miles and he didn't seem to be put off by what I was saying. We finally came to an intersection where I had to take a right to get home while he kept going straight. After we parted ways, I couldn't help but smile. God had allowed this great conversation with a total stranger because I was having a terrific day, despite being in the hospital for 25 days, having cancer and being on chemo. I laughed. What other opportunities would God open up for me in the future?

That's just what I was thinking when the next man passed me on his bike. "Good morning," he said, just like the first guy. "It's a great morning," I shouted. But this one just kept on going. I think I scared him. He never even looked back.

Opportunity

It's hard to think of terminal illness as an opportunity. But there is actually more opportunity in suffering than in comfort. My diagnosis has been a time for me to rearrange my thinking to fit what my purpose in life is supposed to be. That purpose is Jesus. Pure and simple. It's all about him. I want to be known as his friend and tell people about him. They are far more interested in hearing the story of someone in the midst of suffering than to hear about someone in perfect health watching Monday Night Football in their La-Z-Boy.

Recently I was filling my car with gas at 7:15 in the morning when a female attendant wearing a bright green safety vest walked by and greeted me. "Good morning."

"Good morning," I responded with a little wave.

"How are you doing?"

"I'm optimistic."

"Oh, I like that. What are you optimistic about?"

"Well," I said, "I had COVID. I was in the hospital for 25 days and during that time they found out I have cancer. It's not curable but it is treatable." I smiled. "It's been going well so far so I'm really optimistic about the future."

Her expression displayed genuine concern as she listened to my story until at the very end she returned my optimistic smile. "My husband is a cancer survivor too."

"That's wonderful. I'm happy for both of you." We chatted about his cancer journey and then I continued. "I don't know about your husband's experience, but this has really given me time to think about the deeper things. I wouldn't trade it for anything. I'm in a great place. And I get to have great conversations with people like you."

She cocked her head to one side with a curious grin.

The gas nozzle clicked off and I pulled it from the car and put it back on the pump. "Can I leave you with a couple of my favorite verses?" She nodded and took a small step forward. "This is from the end of Psalm 27, verses 13 and 14, "I would have lost heart, unless I had believed that I would see the goodness of the Lord in the land of the living. Wait on the Lord; be of good courage, and He shall strengthen your heart; wait, I say, on the Lord." (NKJV)

"I like that. Thank you."

"Okay, I've gotta give you one more," I chuckled, "and this will be my prayer for you today. It's from Romans 15:13 (NIV)," "May the God of hope fill you with all joy and peace as you trust in him, so that you may overflow with hope by the power of the Holy Spirit."

"Wow," she said, "I gotta write that one down."

God provides opportunities like that all the time and I've learned that everyone is looking for some kind of hope. Many have had family members afflicted with cancer and they're eager to hear from someone with a positive attitude in the middle of the battle. I'll fill them in on my health journey and explain how God has been so good to me through everything. Why wouldn't they want to hear about what God can do for them too? In Psalm 103:2-4 (NIV) David writes, "Praise the Lord, my soul, and forget not all His benefits – who forgives all your sins and heals all your diseases, who redeems your life from the pit and crowns you with love and compassion…" That's what God wants to do for us. Why would my time with COVID and cancer be any different? Every day he crowns me with love and compassion.

I don't know exactly how God uses these conversations in people's lives. They seem encouraged by the scripture I quote, and often the words seem to be a direct message from God to their specific need. I just know that I need to be transparent. If it's out of my heart and based on scripture, then God can use it.

There is more opportunity in suffering than in comfort.

God can use your journey to encourage others. He may bring people to you who are struggling with the same thing you are. You can offer hope because of what you have seen God do in your own life.

Chemo and Red

The oncology team at Mayo decided that six rounds of chemo over six months would be the best way to attack the mantel cell lymphoma. Each treatment would be administered over two consecutive days; the first day's infusions would take several hours, and the second required only an hour or two.

My first round started on February 22nd and I adjusted to it pretty well. I didn't lose my hair and after a couple days of heavy fatigue, I bounced back to my merry old self. There were times when Sharon even forgot that I had cancer.

When I returned to Mayo in March for my next treatment, they ushered me into room #48. It was the second day so the actual infusion would only take about 15 minutes, but they had to mix it up and do a bunch of other stuff so it would take about an hour and a half to two hours.

The room was nice, clinical, but still nice. It was about 10 feet by 10 feet with a reclining chair that vibrates and heats up. It was very comfortable. Then they had the IV tree that they hung all the bags on, a stool for the medical staff, and a curtain if I wanted privacy. But I didn't really want privacy, so I sat there in my heated La-Z-Boy looking out the open door at the nurses station. All of a sudden, I saw a head. I couldn't see where the woman was sitting because she was sideways and perpendicular. Her head popped in and she said, "Hello there. I'll be there. I'm taking care of you today, but I'll be there in just a minute. Okay?" Then she was gone. Her head popped back out of view.

A couple minutes later she walked through the door. She was all of four foot ten inches tall. What she lacked in height, she made up in energy. She bounced around the room, full of life. "My name is, Red." She pointed to her nametag. "See, Red." Then she threw her hair in my face. "See? Red hair. Red," she declared. "That's who I am. I'm going to be taking care of you today and we'll try to get you out of here quickly. So, tell me, how are you feeling?"

"Well, I'm actually feeling pretty good. I'm feeling optimistic, actually. I did wake up at 2:00am this morning because of that steroid they gave me yesterday."

"Oh, yeah, I'm sorry," she said. "Were you able to go back to sleep?"

"Yeah," I said simply.

"Well, what did you do? Did you toss and turn?"

"Truth be told," I said, "those are actually some of my favorite times to wake up."

"Why's that?"

"It gives me an opportunity to talk to God."

She gave me a puzzled but interested expression. "Tell me more."

"I was just lying there. There's nothing else I was going to do at 2:00am so scripture came to mind. My mother taught me a love of the Bible when I was a kid so I memorized verses. A lot of that stuff comes back to me in the middle of the night. I have really great conversations with God.

There was that expression again. "Well, tell me more."

"At two in the morning last night, Psalm 103 came to mind. It's one of my favorite passages to ponder."

"Bless the Lord, oh my soul, and all my inmost being praise His holy name.

Bless the Lord, oh my soul, and forget not all His benefits.

Who forgives all your sins and heals all your diseases,

(Then comes one of my favorite lines.)

Who redeems your life from the pit and crowns you with love and compassion." (NIV)

I proceeded to go through the whole psalm – all 22 verses.

Now she was stopped and just watching me. I realized that

reciting a whole psalm was showing off a bit, but she seemed to be listening so I kept going. When I was done she said, "You aren't going to believe this, but I have to tell you something." She stared hard at me and shook her head slightly. "You aren't going to believe this," she said again and took a deep breath. "I'm a Christian but I'm going through some hard stuff right now. This morning I was talking to God and said, God, I need you to speak to me today." Her eyes took on an even greater intensity. "You're it."

"What do you mean?"

"You're it. You're God's answer to my prayer."

She started crying. I started crying.

Then she started bouncing around again. "Okay, I'm done crying. I'm done crying." She started making some adjustments on the equipment. "Keep talking. I have to do some other stuff here so keep talking."

I quoted some other scripture and we discussed it. She gave me my infusion. Then she started to wrap things up.

I said, "I have a couple of verses I want to leave with you. This is a direct quote from God. It's good stuff. Isaiah 41:10 (NIV) "So do not fear, for I am with you; do not be dismayed, for I am your God. I will strengthen you and help you; I will uphold you with My righteous right hand."

She smiled. "Okay, what else you got?"

"I know that you gotta get going and I gotta get going," I said, "but Psalm 27 is a great passage to think through at two in the morning when the big "what ifs" pop into your head. The boogey men get bigger and scarier in the middle of the night. But what happens is this – when you look at scripture, the "what ifs" and the boogey men come face-to-face with the Great I Am.

I'll give you just the last two verses of Psalm 27," I said. "This is for both of us today." "I would have lost heart, unless I had believed that I would see the goodness of the Lord in the land of the living. Wait on the Lord; be of good courage, and He shall strengthen your heart; wait, I say, on the Lord." (NKJV)

Red arched her eyebrows. "Wow." Then she ran out of the room to take care of another patient. About three minutes later she came back in and said, "You're not going to believe this." She cocked her head thoughtfully to one side. "That last verse you just gave me, that's exactly what they needed to hear in the next room." She began to tear up but quickly wiped her eyes. "I'm not going to cry again. I'm not crying. I'm fine."

I smiled and said, "Red, it might not be here, but I will see you again. I'll see you again."

♦

Sometimes you can be the answer to someone else's prayer, even in the middle of your own trial. Are you open to seeing and meeting the needs of others when you are still waiting for God to meet your own?

On Assignment

Many years ago, I had a building contractor friend with a deep faith that showed not only in his work, but also in his attitude. When I asked him about it, he told me that the first thing he prays every morning is, "God, it's me, reporting for duty. What's my assignment today?" He relies on God to lead him through his day: to the people he should talk to and the things he should accomplish.

I realize that it's a very simple declaration of trust and commitment, but I love it. That's the frame of mind that I have today. *God, it's John, reporting for duty. What's my assignment?* And it's clear what God has assigned me at this point in time. Get the treatments. Do what the doctors tell me to do. Trust God to fill in the blanks. Then, look for the opportunities that he gives me to talk to people. They can come at the most unexpected times.

Recently, I was on a call with a man whose company provides a service to insurance firms like mine. I had never met him personally, but I'm guessing from his voice that he's in his mid-forties.

Making small talk, he started with, "What's going on with you? Have you been busy?"

Most of the time, those kinds of questions are just pleasantries and they don't really care about the answer. You're busy. I'm busy. We're all busy. And that's as far as it goes. But this guy asked me a couple of times, so I thought, *Well, if you really want to know…* I proceeded to tell him about the 25 days in the hospital with COVID and how it led to other tests and the discovery of cancer.

I think he was a bit dumbstruck. The discussion had taken a sudden hard left turn that he didn't expect, but I could tell he was interested.

I blurted out the whole story about the richness of my experience, life and eternity, and the one monkey that everyone on planet earth carries on their back: we're all going to die. Everybody knows that.

I explained to him that over the last few months I had the chance to think more about God. I told him about inviting Jesus into my heart at age five and that it was a good experience. When my mother presented it to me, she talked about Hell and I knew I didn't want to go there. Then later in college, I started to figure out what I really believed. I believed in intelligent design. I believed in the Bible and what it says about Jesus.

He seemed to be interested in my story so I went on. I told

him that recently I'd been thinking about how God created everything perfect. He said it was good. Then sin entered the world and messed it up. It's a genetic thing. We all have it. We have a propensity to sin.

To me, the whole Bible is the story of God reaching out to us saying, "You're all sick. You have a problem and I have the remedy for it."

I explained that Hell is an option. People don't have to go there. In fact, God didn't create Hell for us. He made it for Satan and the demons who rebelled against him. It just so happens that anyone who wants to follow in their tracks gets to go there too. But you don't have to. We're all in desperate straits and God is continually throwing the lifeline out to us. God is patient. God is kind. God is waiting.

He started to compare Christianity to other religions but I don't think he was trying to put me off. I'm sure he was just processing everything. I'm willing to bet that he'd never had a business call talking about Heaven, Hell, God, judgment, Jesus, sin and repentance. Then he said, "I know there's something bigger out there."

I couldn't help but smile on my end of the line. "God made you that way," I said. "He made you with a God-shaped vacuum in there telling you there's got to be more than this. And God is saying to you, I'm it. I want to fill you with a relationship with me."

By the time we finished talking, I'm sure the guy's hair was blown back from everything he'd heard. I thought later, *You idiot. You did all the talking. Why didn't you ask him more questions?* But it seemed like the Holy Spirit responded to me. *Don't you worry about that. You don't even know which things you said might make a difference. You gave me plenty of material that I can work with on this guy.*

It reminded me that even though I'd like to get better at articulating the Gospel message, we don't save anybody ourselves. The Holy Spirit does that. He does the work and we're just the tellers.

I wrapped up the phone call by saying, "This conversation started with us talking about some insurance questions. That was the deal. But I've come to understand that the deal is not the deal. It really wasn't about that. We only spent a half hour on that. The real deal was the sidebar issue. The real deal was about life. You're not a body with a soul. You're a soul with a body. The body is going to go away but your soul is going to live forever. The question is, what's the address going to be?"

I enjoy being on assignment. I never know what opportunities God has planned for me.

God, it's John, reporting for duty. What's my assignment?

---◆---

Are you on assignment for God today?

Make yourself available for the conversations God opens for you.

Try praying, God it's (name), reporting for duty. What's my assignment? Then look for the opportunities he gives you to talk to people. They may come at the most unexpected times.

From the Mind of God

My wife, Sharon, and I were waiting on an elevator at the Mayo Clinic after one of my chemo treatments and this lady with a big fur coat came over. She was probably around eighty years old and, from her wardrobe, looked like she had some money. The doors opened and the three of us stepped into the elevator. We started up a conversation and it wasn't long before she asked, "Where are you from?"

"From the mind of God," I blurted out.

Her head snapped around fast enough to give her whiplash. All she could do was look at me and wonder what was going to come out of my mouth next.

I thought about it afterwards and realized that it was a really strange thing to say, but it was the absolute truth. He's known me before the existence of time. All my days were ordained by him. I didn't think myself up. God did.

Therefore, I did come from the mind of God.

Our friend in the fur coat said she was at Mayo first for cancer and then they found a heart issue. After we parted ways, we saw her trying to light a cigarette as she walked down the street in a stiff breeze. Go figure.

I know my answer to her question was strange, but I guarantee that she thought about it later. Maybe I didn't give the Holy Spirit a lot of material to work with, but it's what I had at the moment.

A Possibility of Hope

After only two rounds of chemo, the doctor ordered another PET scan to check my progress. Sharon and dozens of others had been praying for me, so hopes were high that the scan would be clear. Sharon, of course, prayed for complete healing. I, on the other hand, tend to go into these meetings a little more detached, with few expectations, knowing that whatever God wants to happen, will happen.

In late March, we traveled to Mayo to hear the news.

"What do you think the results of your PET scan were?" The doctor asked.

Sharon knew immediately that it must be good news or he wouldn't have started that way. She squeezed my hand extra hard and her eyes sparkled with renewed hope.

The doctor held up an 8.5 x 11 inch print of the scan from January. "You see all the active hot spots in the liver and the lymph nodes?" He pointed to multiple sites where the cancer had been active and growing. Sharon and I had seen it before and nodded silently. Then he held up the latest scan. "Look here. None of those spots are on the new PET scan." I felt a strong squeeze on my hand from Sharon again. "We still have that one-inch mass in your lung, but it hasn't grown since we last looked at it. We'll have to do a biopsy at some point but, for now, it's not growing and that's good."

Sharon and I sat in a stunned silence, but not for long.

"Sharon, what did you expect?" the doctor asked.

"I expected all of it to be gone."

He chuckled, "That's asking a lot of only two rounds of chemo."

"John, how about you?"

"I was just hoping to make some kind of progress. I've never done this before."

The doctor chuckled again and then shook my hand with a grip strong enough to break my wrist. I know he had to maintain some kind of professional decorum, but I could tell he was pleased with the results.

Before we could leave the clinic, we had to stop by the pharmacy for a prescription. I struck up a conversation with the pharmacist, and I told her that the whole treatment process had been fascinating and I was having the best time of my life.

"How can you say that?" She asked.

I said, "Jesus' half-brother told us to consider it all joy when you fall into various tests."

Sharon noticed the pharmacist had a blank stare on her face and we quickly moved on to another topic. I doubt if most people quote scripture and talk about Jesus' half-brother when they're waiting for their prescriptions.

On our way home, we stopped for lunch at a place that has the world's best lemonade. As we sunk into the cushioned leather seats, breathing in the savory aromas coming off the grill, and taking a deep drink of the tart lemonade, the tension of our clinical morning melted away. The reality of my new prognosis slowly began to seep into our consciousness. This was really good news. There was reason for hope. We now had permission to think past the next few weeks and make plans for our future.

When we got back home to Minneapolis there were still the everyday details of life to attend to. Our move to Florida was fast approaching, and I needed more packing boxes so I stopped at Home Depot.

It was quiet when I walked through the door and a young woman in her mid-twenties greeted me. "Hi, welcome to Home Depot. How are you today?"

"I'm optimistic."

"Really?" She asked. "That's great. What are you optimistic about?"

Not many people ask me that, but just as I was getting ready to answer, someone came to check out and I said, "I'll wait for you to finish. You go ahead and help them."

When she was done I told her, "I was diagnosed with cancer a while back and I just went to see my doctor today. The test results came back showing that the cancer is apparently not obvious."

"Oh, can I give you a hug?" she asked, and I gave her a big hug.

Then somebody else came to check out. I said, "I need to get some boxes. I'll come back and tell you more."

When I returned, her eyes were bright and her smile was inviting. "That's great news."

"I thank Jesus for that," I said. "I really do."

She glanced around, maybe looking for more interruptions from customers or checking to see if her supervisor was watching. "I have to tell you something," she said. "A little while ago I was going to do some things that I really shouldn't be doing. But I was going to do them anyway. Then my sister came into my room one night and asked if I was alright. She wanted to know if there was something going on that I needed to talk about." Her eyes misted over. "She came at just the right time and it prevented me from doing it. I realize that I need to get ahold of my life now."

I returned her smile. "Let me give you a verse." I recited Isaiah 41:10 (NIV). "So do not fear, for I am with you; do not be dismayed, for I am your God. I will strengthen you and help you; I will uphold you with My righteous right hand."

"Oh, that's good," she said. "Can I share a verse with you?"

"Sure."

"Consider the lilies, how they grow: they neither toil nor spin; and yet I say to you, even Solomon in all his glory was not arrayed like one of these. If then God so clothes the grass, which today is in the field and tomorrow is thrown into the oven, how much more will He clothe you, O you of little faith? (Luke 12:27,28 NKJV) "I just love that verse."

"It's such a great verse," I said. "You don't have to worry. God will provide."

I finally had to check out and head home. "Can you tell me your name?"

"It's Kathy."

"Well, Kathy, my name's John. It's been great to talk with you. I have to tell you that you have a Jesus shine on your face today. I can see that."

"Aww," she blushed a little. "You just made my day."

"I know what a Jesus shine looks like because my daughter has that. She sparkles and you've got that too."

"Wow," she said, smiling brightly while her eyes misted up again.

I got in my car and took off toward home but started laughing on the way. I had come into the store feeling really good about my day. I knew I should be looking for opportunities to talk to people, but I really didn't feel like it. Then Kathy happened and it just made me laugh about what God has in mind. There are so many opportunities to encourage people if we can just engage with them.

I laughed all the way home. Then I told Sharon all about it. We watched a little TV and went to bed early. I woke up at 2:00am like I often do, but it wasn't because of worry. I was still laughing at how God works. With a happy grin on my face, I turned over to go back to a very peaceful sleep. *God, I can't believe all this stuff you're doing.*

I didn't dare look at a clock again. *I've got to get back to sleep,* I thought. *I can't get behind on my sleep. I'll be in trouble.* But I was so full of praise and thankfulness to the Lord. I laughed at all the little vignettes that he's brought me into. It was just amazing. It made me think again of coming through a fog-filled forest and bursting out into a clearing of bright sunshine and all kinds of beauty that I've never experienced before. I was right where God wanted me.

Has God given you reason for hope in the middle of a difficult situation?

Be confident of God's good plans for you.

Little Bunny and the Big Bad Giant

I was lying in bed when a crash above me sounded like someone had dropped an ironing board. I looked around and listened, but there was nothing more. It was quiet again.

I was in the basement of my daughter's house enjoying some quiet time before everyone else in the house woke up. But the quiet was suddenly interrupted again with another loud clatter above my head. I opened the curtain of the egress window next to the bed and there on the other side of the glass was a very frightened little bunny who had fallen into the pit. He ran in panicked circles around the four-foot-wide window well and jumped erratically toward the blue sky and freedom that were just out of his reach.

I confess that my first thought may have been to get a brick from the garage, hit it over the head, and bury it in the backyard. Then it occurred to me that I was in the position of asking God for a lot of mercy right now. Maybe I should show a little mercy to this bunny. But how?

I went to the garage, not to look for a brick, but to find a board for the little critter to climb up like a ladder. Nothing I found was long enough. Then I saw my daughter's gardening gloves. I thought I could go down into the window well, pick up the rabbit and lift it out. Simple. But my mind was suddenly filled with scenes of the killer rabbit from *Monty Python and the Holy Grail* and I worried about keeping my head attached to my body.

Forcing those images from my mind, I donned the gloves and climbed down the ladder. The terrified little creature looked up at me with big brown eyes, knowing with certainty in his little bunny brain that I was coming down to destroy him.

My foot hit the gravel at the bottom of the window well as the bunny cowered against the far wall. Slowly I reached out to grab him but he broke into a panicked run, hopping madly with nowhere to go. I spun in circles trying to get ahold of him, but each time I grabbed for him, he hopped out of reach and I was left with nothing but air or the momentary hold of a back leg. Finally, I anticipated his next hop and I got my hands around him, but he wriggled and kicked for all he was worth and got away again. I realized that to hang on to him, I would have to squeeze him so tight I would crush his little body.

The two of us stood staring at each other on opposite sides of the window well. He was terrified and I was frustrated and perplexed about what to do.

Suddenly, he jumped straight up and he almost reached the top of the window well. Then he jumped a second time and again he was almost to the lip of the wall and the freedom he so desper ately desired. I watched absolutely mystified. Then the third time he jumped, the thought occurred to me, *I'll just give him a little boost at the top of his jump.* And it worked! He jumped. I scooped him up and over the edge of the wall onto the grass. He hopped a safe distance away. Then before he disappeared into the bushes, he looked back over his shoulder at me as if to say, "Hey, you touched my butt!"

I stood there five feet deep in the window well just laughing. It made me think of God's mercy to us. How many wonderful things does he do for us or try to do for us that we don't know about? We're afraid. We don't let him help us. Just like the bunny, we see God coming down into our world to destroy us or mess up our lives. We don't recognize the rescue that he's offering.

There is a verse in Psalm 18:29 (NIV) where David says, "With Your help I can advance against a troop; with my God I can scale a wall." I realized that, just like the bunny, we need to do the jumping and God will do the lifting.

---◆---

Reflect on the many wonderful things God does for you every day.

Is there some event that you may have seen as negative that God is actually using for a positive outcome in your life?

Have you witnessed God "lifting" you up at a critical moment when you couldn't do it on your own?

God's Kindness

As I read through the Gospels, I'm amazed at all the kind things Jesus did for people. He healed the sick. He restored sight to the blind. He spent time with the rejected of society. He cared for widows and small children. He even provided wine for a wedding celebration.

He didn't preach to people right away. I think that's what drew people to him. Sure, he had harsh words for the religious hypocrites, but for the everyday down-and-out slugs like you and me, he was kind and loving. No wonder large crowds followed him.

I think if we were to examine our own lives, we would recognize evidence of his daily kindness to us. One recent example in my cancer story happened on the morning of June 2nd. I had just had a chemo treatment Thursday morning at Mayo Clinic in Minnesota. I needed to have a follow-up injection twenty-four hours later, but we really didn't want to wait around another day for just one more shot. The nurses fitted me with a wearable abdominal injection device that was programmed to give me my medication at precisely the right time on Friday so we could return to Florida.

I went to bed that night feeling the normal fatigue that comes after every chemo treatment. I was looking forward to a good night's sleep, but as I sat on the edge of the bed, I glanced down at the injection device on my stomach. A little red warning light was blinking.

I had been told that if that happened, the device was not working properly and to call my provider immediately. So much for the start of a restful night's sleep.

I put a call in to the clinic and a nurse told me that it was possible the device might still deliver my medication as scheduled. They couldn't remotely determine what was causing the malfunction. In any case, I could expect a call first thing the next morning with further instructions.

I sat back down again on the edge of the bed looking at the phone in my hand. I desperately wanted to go to sleep, but I had another issue. Every day I received an encouraging text message from a retired pastor friend. Since it was automated, I had no way of knowing when it would be delivered. I didn't want to be awakened, but I also didn't want to shut off my phone and risk missing the call from Mayo. I sat for a minute and considered my options. For the sake of uninterrupted sleep, I silenced my phone.

I woke up late the next morning and glanced at the time, somewhat concerned. Florida is one hour ahead of Minnesota so I thought that Mayo might call at any moment. I was still groggy, half awake and half asleep, just wanting to lay there for a while. But there was an emphatic nudge of my spirit to turn on my phone. Just as I picked it up, the screen told me a call was coming in from area code 507, Rochester Minnesota. It was the consulting nurse from Mayo.

It may not have been a parting-of-the-Red-Sea kind of miracle, but to me it was just another example of God's kindness. I was able to get a full night of uninterrupted sleep and then God nudged me awake just in time to answer my phone.

Ephesians 2: 6-7 (NIV)

"And God raised us up with Christ and seated us with Him in the heavenly realms in Christ Jesus, in order that in the coming ages He might show the incomparable riches of His grace, expressed in His **kindness** to us in Christ Jesus."

◆

God's everyday miracles can be mistaken for coincidence. How have you experienced God's kindness in the middle of your trial?

Mantel Cell Lymphoma is Gone

As a cancer patient, one thing you never want to see is your oncologist scrunch his face up and frown when he's analyzing your test results. But that's what happened after my June 27th PET scan. "There's a whole bunch of stuff here that I wasn't expecting to see," he said. "I want to order a bronchoscopy, a biopsy of the lymph nodes and one of that mass in your lung."

Our emotions were thrown back into the fire. What did this mean? Last month the doctor had been so encouraging after my last scan. The cancer hotspots that had been growing and active in January were now extinguished and supposedly not an issue. We even held out hope that I wouldn't need to go through more chemo. Now this. But I knew that God was still faithful.

The bronchoscopy was scheduled for Tuesday, July 5th, and I sailed through it. I didn't even have a sore throat. Then Sharon and I drove from Rochester up to our cabin in Northern Minnesota. My next appointment was scheduled for just three days later, even though the doctor said the tests would take a full five days. At 1:15 we were sitting in front of his desk when he came into the room shaking his head. "I'm sorry to say that we don't have the results of the tests back yet so I guess we'll talk about what we've got so far."

Just then his computer chimed telling him that the test results were in. Instead of five days, the results came back in three and a half. He took a moment to review them and then looked back up at us. "The mantel cell lymphoma isn't an issue anymore," he declared. Sharon and I stole a hopeful look at each other. He didn't use words like cured or remission, but he definitely said we didn't need to do anything more with it. No Chemo. No surgery. No nothing.

"But there is this adenoma in your right lung that we need to check on."

"Are you the guy for that," I asked.

"No, you need to see another specialist in the clinic."

Great. I was thinking, *it's Friday afternoon at the Mayo Clinic. What are the chances of getting an appointment with another busy oncologist?* The doctor came back into the room a few minutes later and said, "I have an appointment set up for you within the hour with a specialist in the lung cancer area." God surprised us again.

A few minutes later we were sitting in front of another desk talking with Dr. Marx. I asked him if he had any brothers who made movies back in the thirties and forties. He must have heard that joke before because he just smirked and shook his head.

"I need to find out a lot more about this mass in your lung. I need to see the biopsy and I want to do some other tests on you. I won't really know until I see all that." Then he asked a lot of questions including whether I was a smoker.

"I never smoked. I've never even tried it," I said. "But I have been around a lot of campfires."

He smirked again, "I don't know if it's surgery we're looking at or chemo and radiation. If you've never smoked, but you still have cancer in that lung, there could be something genetic causing the cancer. If that's the case, we can treat it with a pill."

"I vote for that one," I said.

◆

Your hope may be up one minute and down the next. What verses do you cling to when the roller coaster of diagnosis and treatment take your emotions for a ride?

God's peace can fill you at any time, no matter what outcome you may face.

The Boogeyman Defeated...again

I woke with a start and looked around the room. The only light came from the soft glow of a beside clock telling me it was 2:30 in the morning. I heard Sharon's gentle breathing next to me and was relieved she was still asleep. Often when I wake up in the middle of the night, my mind slowly comes to consciousness and, eventually, I realize that I've started thinking through issues. Tonight, however, I awoke fully alert with my mind already engaged in processing the latest prognosis.

What was I supposed to make of all this? On one hand, it was great news. The mantel cell lymphoma was dealt with. I didn't need any more treatments. But, on the other hand, there was this other thing, this very ominous sounding thing – lung cancer. I heard those words and I pictured the Marlboro Man, all macho, saddled on his horse, herding longhorns, and coughing up a lung. Was I the Marlboro Man? Even as I laid in bed, I shook my head at the absurd thought. An involuntary shiver ran up my spine as the icy fingers of fear tried to grab ahold of me again.

I sighed, reminding myself, *Okay, what do I have to do again? That's right. I have to trust God.* I ran through the drill. *What's the first 'T'? Oh, yeah, Give Thanks.*

1 Thessalonians 5:18 (NKJV) "...in everything give thinks for this is the will of God in Christ Jesus for you."

The ceiling reflected the faintest red glow from the clock. I tried to stare past it, applying the meaning of the verse to my life once again. *Okay, what am I thankful for?*

I'm thankful that the mantel cell lymphoma is dealt with. That's pretty good.

What else? Well, when you're at war and you're in a foxhole with your buddy, it binds you together in special ways that you wouldn't normally be bound. I'm kind of in a foxhole fighting a war against cancer and God is in here with me. What a great way to get to know him better. Okay, I'm thankful for that too.

Now my eyes were wide open and my mind was firing on all cylinders thinking of all the things I had to be thankful for. I glanced at Sharon still breathing softly beside me, pushed back the covers and swung my feet to the floor. I had to get up to write these things down. They were too good to forget in the morning. I went to my desk in the other room, turned on the lamp, and pulled out a notebook and pen, hurrying to capture my thoughts.

Things to be thankful for:

1. Answered prayer. Mantel cell is in remission. I remember telling people that if I don't die from mantel cell, I'll die from something else. Well, voila, God has taken care of me with mantel cell, so now I can die of something else.

2. Enhanced relationship with God. What better way is there to get to know someone than to work together on a common project, like being in a foxhole together fighting a common enemy? Psalm 23:4 (NKJV) says "Yea, though I walk through the valley of the shadow of death, I will fear no evil: for You are with me…" and Psalm 91:15 (NKJV) "He shall call upon me, and I will answer him; I will be with him in trouble; I will deliver him and honor him." God promises to go through this with me. How great is that?

3. I acknowledge that eventually I am going to die. Here's how David described it in 1 Kings 2:2 (NKJV) "I go the way of all the earth…" That's a little smoother than saying, I'm going to die. But until that day, and including that day, I acknowledge that God is in full control. Psalm 31:15 (NKJV) "My times are in Your hand…" Psalm 18:30 (NKJV) "As for God, His way is perfect…" Psalm 115:3 (NKJV) "But our God is in heaven; He does whatever He pleases."

4. "The Lord is my helper." Hebrews 13:6 (NIV) and Deuteronomy 31:6 (NIV) "…He will never leave you nor forsake you." I thought about how God had been my helper. The test results that were supposed to take at least five days arrived two days early, while we were sitting in the doctor's office. Then it was discovered I have a different kind of cancer and need to see another specialist. Viola! An appointment was arranged within the hour on a busy Friday afternoon.

Without the Lord, one would be compelled to use words like "coincidence" or "lucky" instead of looking at it from the biblical view of Romans 8:28. "And we know that all things work together for good to those who love God, to those who are called according to His purpose." (NKJV)

5. Miracles. God has performed miracles in the past, and he has not changed. He still performs miracles today. Hebrews 13:8 (NKJV) "Jesus Christ is the same yesterday, today and forever." Psalm 103:2-4 (NIV) "Praise the Lord, my soul, and forget not all His benefits – Who forgives your sins and heals all your diseases, Who redeems your life from the pit and crowns you with love and compassion…"

God knows my name and he hasn't changed. He is a miracle-working God.

6. "Dead men don't praise God. You can't testify once you're dead." That's the John Whaley paraphrase of Psalm 30:9. And Psalm 34:2 (NKJV) says, "My soul shall make its boast in the Lord…"

It made me think. Those who die quietly in their sleep aren't able to speak of God's goodness to those left behind. It's those of us going through the trials who get to talk about all the good stuff God does. James 1:2 (NIV) says, "Consider it pure joy, my brothers and sisters, whenever you face trials of many kinds…"

Not only do I get the benefit of refinement by trials, but I also get to tell people about God's goodness and provision for me in the trial.

Trials magnify the greatness of God.

1 Thessalonians 5:18 – That little verse got my mind off of my problems and onto the problem solver. I was tired. I was emotionally worn out, but that verse turned me around to think about things I was thankful for. It opened up a whole world of optimistic possibility. What started with fear and anxiety at 2:30 in the morning, soon became a delightful encounter with the Holy Spirit – and a return to peaceful sleep.

◆

When fear strikes in the middle of the night, you can consciously decide to be thankful in the midst of your circumstances.

Here is a place to start:

• What prayers have you seen answered?

• How has your relationship with God grown deeper during this trial?

• Have you witnessed God's presence and help in your circumstances?

• How has he used your situation to encourage others?

When you face fear:

• Do you acknowledge that God is still in complete control?

• Do you believe that God is still a God of miracles?

• What big life-changing miracles and/or small everyday miracles have you experienced?

It's those of us going through the trials who get to talk about all the good stuff God does.

Oh, by the Way, You Have Brain Cancer

All attention for my medical treatment shifted dramatically after my July 5th bronchoscopy and biopsy. Mantel cell lymphoma was no longer an issue, but lung cancer loomed large in our sights. The pulmonologist at Mayo wanted one more round of scans before making my treatment plan. On July 15th, I was scheduled for a chest PET scan, a full lung function test, and then a brain scan to make sure the cancer hadn't snuck anywhere else in my body.

I flew in early the day before for a required COVID test. After a quick nostril swab and temperature scan, the remainder of the day was mine. I left Mayo and drove about forty miles through the scenic bluffs of Southeastern Minnesota to the pretty little town of Lanesboro along the Root River. After grabbing a bite to eat, I sat down on the grassy bank of the river to watch the water meander downstream. I've always loved water, and looking out at it that day seemed to calm and nourish my soul. The towering elms and cottonwoods lining the banks shaded me from the midsummer sun and a breeze blowing off the water cooled my face. It was the perfect place to pause and pray and thank God again for all he was doing. I could feel my heartbeat and breathing begin to relax. I could also sense God's presence with me there. It was the perfect preparation for my upcoming day of medical tests and the troubling news that would soon follow.

After my chest PET scan and a brain scan the next morning, I had five hours to kill before returning for a full lung function test in the afternoon. I was halfway back to the clinic when I got a call from the doctor. I'd learned by then that any time a doctor calls back too soon after a test, it's probably not good news. "John," he said, "we already got the results of the brain scan back and we detected two spots where cancer has appeared."

My breath caught in my throat. I was taken totally by surprise. No one had even mentioned the possibility of brain cancer. "That sounds serious," I said.

"Yes," he stated, "it is a serious thing. It's not so threatening now. The spots of cancer are very small right now, about the size of the point of a pen, but if you don't do anything, it'll get serious pretty quickly."

I let out the breath I'd been holding. "Okay, what do we do?"

"There's a procedure called gamma knife surgery that I would recommend. It uses focused gamma rays coming from multiple angles to attack and kill the cancer cells deep in your brain. It won't affect the healthy cells surrounding the cancer. It's extremely precise."

"How long will I be in the hospital?"

"That's the amazing thing about this surgery," he said. "It's an outpatient treatment. You'll be in and out of here within half a day. Mayo has done over ten thousand surgeries like this. It's been very successful. There's nothing to worry about."

And just like that, I was scheduled for brain surgery on July 27th.

I flew back to Florida that night and gave Sharon the scary news. Just the mention of brain cancer was a sobering thought for both of us.

A few days later I met with an oncologist in Florida for a second opinion. He examined my scans and concurred with everything the doctors at Mayo suggested. He also gave us a new reason for hope. I had been classified by the doctors at Mayo as having stage four cancer because it had already spread to other parts of my body. But this doctor said, "You're really more like stage three because these little spots in your brain are so small right now. The question you need to ask your doctors at Mayo is how would they treat your cancer differently if it was stage three instead of four?"

Both Sharon and I left his office with renewed optimism that we were heading in the right direction and starting to see the results we were hoping for.

On July 27th, less than two weeks after my diagnosis, I underwent gamma knife brain surgery. It went even better than the doctor described. Including preparation and the complete procedure, I was only there for three hours. Pain free. Two small spots of cancer were obliterated and no others were detected.

Mantel cell lymphoma – Check

Brain cancer – Check

The cancer kept popping up but we kept knocking it down. I was starting to feel like a human whack-a-mole.

◆

It's hard to fight off discouragement when it seems all Hell is breaking out against you and your situation is getting worse.

How have you seen God's faithfulness in your circumstances?

Praying for Healing

I would love for the cancer to be taken away, but I don't feel an overwhelming sadness about it one way or the other. I confess that I'm not even really praying for healing right now. I might be in denial or I may not be wanting to set myself up for disappointment.

Some people say, *pray aggressively*. Don't say, *if it's your will,* because then you have an out. Pray believing. But Jesus prayed, *if it be your will.* I recognize that I know very little about how God works, but I know he does.

On the other hand, I know that many people are praying for me, people I don't even know, and that humbles me. For example, I go to a Tuesday morning Bible study in Fort Myers. There are about 5 to 15 guys who meet at Panera Bread at 7:00am, as soon as it opens. This particular week, we were talking about James, chapter 5. Each man shared his observation of a particular verse and how it might apply to them.

We had gotten about halfway around the table when it was my friend, Jesús', turn. He picked verses 14 and 15. "Is anyone among you sick? Then he must call for the elders of the church and they are to pray over him, anointing him with oil in the name of the Lord; and the prayer of faith will restore the one who is sick…" (NIV) After reading the verses he looked around the table at the other men. "Why don't we do this?" he said. "We have a brother here who is sick. Why don't we pray for him and anoint him with oil right now?"

I looked over at Jesús and my eyes grew a little wider and I sat up a little straighter.

One man quickly left the table. I wasn't sure where he was going, but the others rose from their chairs and gathered around me. Before they could start praying, the first man came back with a little cup of olive oil he'd gotten from the front counter. They poured the oil over my blonde Finlander hair, laid hands on me, and Jesús prayed for my healing. Eight men stood and prayed for me right there in the middle of Panera Bread. It was amazing. I'd never experienced anything like that. I didn't necessarily feel the electricity of restored health, but my tear ducts, that are rarely used and virtually new, started to leak a little. It was a powerful time of encouragement and love shown by my Christian friends.

A few days later, we had an electrician come to the house. We needed him to wire and install a ceiling fan in our living room. Carlos came to the door with his assistant and handed me his card. On the back, in very small lettering, was printed "Philippians 4:13," the reference for the Bible verse, "I can do all things through Christ who strengthens me." (NKJV) I've been burned by other supposed Christian businessmen who use Bible verses and Christian terms for marketing, so I waited to see if Carlos was really a man of faith.

In the first few minutes as he and his assistant were analyzing the project, his attention was drawn to a picture on the wall. The painting depicts Joseph's workshop with young Jesus playing on the floor with three long iron spikes. Bright sunlight streaming through a window falls on Jesus and casts the unmistakable shadow of a cross on the floor. Carlos straightened up, "I like that," he said.

I nodded my head. "Yeah, it's a painting of Jesus."

Carlos looked back at the painting again, cocking his head to the side. "I gave my heart to Jesus nine years ago." A gentle smile came to his face and then he bent down to pick up his tools. "I'll tell you about it after I'm done with the job."

It probably took all of 45 minutes for them to finish the work. Then his assistant went out to the truck while Carlos started to tell us the amazing story of his transformation in Christ. He had come from Cuba where he was addicted to alcohol, drugs, sex, and anything else you could think of. Then Jesus got ahold of him and changed everything. Now, he's an electrician but also an evangelist. He travels all over the world telling people about Jesus.

He told us a story about doing some work at a house where a man sat watching them the whole time they were working. When Carlos was done, he said to the man, "I sense that there's something wrong with you physically, some health issue."

The man replied, "Yeah, I'm going to the doctor tomorrow to have my leg amputated. There's no circulation in it."

"Do you mind if I pray for you?" Carlos asked.

The man nodded and Carlos proceeded to pray. Then he packed up his tools and left and didn't have any further contact with the man until about three weeks later when he returned to the house for some additional work. To his amazement, the man was walking with a cane and his leg was still intact.

"What happened?"

The man grinned. "I went to the doctor and he said we don't need to amputate anymore. There's circulation in the leg now."

Carlos turned to me with a warm smile and an intensity in his eyes, and asked if he could pray for my healing. I confess, my mind flashed immediately to the story he had just told and I wondered if God would do the same for me. Carlos put a hand on my right lung and we had a little prayer meeting right there.

Any electrician could have come to our house that day to do the work, but God sent Carlos – electrician and true man of faith – to pray for me. It was remarkable.

The retired pastor friend I mentioned in chapter 15 experienced a miraculous healing himself from a serious lung disease about 25 years ago. Today, he keeps a list of people he prays for and sends each of us an encouraging text every day. A typical message goes something like this. "Terrific Tuesday to you! Praying for God's complete healing in your life and that your day is full of miracles and God sightings. Love you guys!"

While I'm not sure of my healing yet, it struck me recently that I've been more aware of God's everyday love, kindness and tenderness. Why should I be surprised? I've got my pastor friend specifically praying that for me every day.

So I return to one of my opening thoughts in this chapter. I know very little about how God works – but I know that he does. Mark 11:22-24 (NIV) says, "Have faith in God," Jesus answered. "Truly I tell you, if anyone says to this mountain, 'Go, throw yourself into the sea,' and does not doubt in their heart but believes that what they say will happen, it will be done for them.

Therefore I tell you, whatever you ask for in prayer, believe that you have received it, and it will be yours."

If that's all we had to go on, it would be pretty good. But there is no vending-machine god. This is a relationship and God has his own will. I fit in to his plan, not the other way around. Even in the garden, Jesus asked for something outside of God's will. "O My Father, if it is possible, let this cup pass from Me; nevertheless, not as I will, but as You will." (Matthew 26:39 NKJV) God said "no," and Jesus submitted.

We're told to pray. And prayer makes a difference. It changes things. But a lot of times we say our prayers and don't leave any room for God's sovereignty. The Bible is filled with stories of sick and suffering people who were healed, and many others who were not. There is no formula to getting God to do what we want him to do. There is only trust that God is working all things for our ultimate good and his glory.

◆

The Bible tells us to ask, seek and knock, expecting God to answer our prayers. As you pray:
- Trust that God is working. Pray believing
- Submit to his sovereignty

Fear and Discouragement

The devil does his best work in fear and discouragement. Either one will immobilize us and make us ineffective and unproductive, both in our knowledge of the Lord and in working with people. It's even worse at 2:00 in the morning when you are startled awake by terrifying thoughts echoing in your head with no immediate answers. That's the vulnerability I have. There are some things that could be very scary right now, but I choose not to go there.

If there's a discouraging word or a fearful boogeyman on the horizon, I realize I need to pay attention immediately and stop it in its tracks before it controls my thoughts and emotions. When something bad wakes me in the middle of the night, I start calling scripture to mind to readjust my focus on things above. Isaiah 41:10 (NIV) says, "So do not fear, for I am with you; do not be dismayed, for I am your God. I will strengthen you and help you; I will uphold you with My righteous right hand."

"Fear not." God doesn't promise to take away our fear. Instead, he commands us *not to fear* or be discouraged. He would not have told us to *fear not* if we couldn't *fear not*. I don't know about you, but it isn't always easy to shut off the faucet of fear and discouragement when the spigot is wide open. It can be such a slippery slope. My panicked thoughts tell me that the chemo is going to make me really sick. It's probably not going to work. I'm just going to die anyway. My thoughts can quickly drag me down to the pit of fear and discouragement.

I have to stop myself. Those thoughts are from the enemy, whereas God tells us in 2 Timothy 1:7 (NLT) "For God has not given us a spirit of fear and timidity, but of power, love, and self-discipline." Having a disciplined mind means that I take charge of those thoughts that are coming into my influence. If they are fearful and come from the enemy, I dismiss them. Otherwise, I would be influenced by every boogeyman who pokes his face in my window.

In Psalm 34:6 (NIV) David's experience sounds a lot like mine. "This poor man called, and the Lord heard him; He saved him out of all his troubles." David points out the key for us. Instead of wallowing in fear and discouragement, we're invited to cry out to the Lord. Pour out our hearts. 1 Peter 5:7 (NKJV) instructs us. "casting all your cares upon Him for He cares for you."

Once our hearts are crying out to God, then we can readjust our focus from what the boogeyman would have us believe, to what God wants us to think about. "Finally, brothers and sisters, whatever is true, whatever is noble, whatever is right, whatever is pure, whatever is lovely, whatever is admirable—if anything is excellent or praiseworthy—think about such things." Philippians 4:8 (NIV).

"...we take captive every thought to make it obedient to Christ." 2 Corinthians 10:5 (NIV)

"Set your mind on things above, not on earthly things." Colossians 3:2 (NIV)

"Do not conform to the pattern of this world, but be transformed by the renewing of your mind. Then you will be able to test and approve what God's will is – His good, pleasing and perfect will." Romans 12:2 (NIV)

If you're looking for a formula to follow, Paul says in Romans 12:12 (NIV), "Be joyful in hope, patient in affliction, faithful in prayer." Put that on a bumper sticker as something to live by.

Many years ago, long before my health problems, I did a study on what the Bible says about fear. I don't remember the number exactly, but there was something like 450 verses that mention fear. Approximately half of them instruct us to fear God and obey his commandments. The other half say *fear not.*

What that told me was that we do have fear in this life. The object of my fear is the important thing. My heavenly father is bigger than anything else going on in my life. If I have a healthy fear and reverence for him, then I don't have to be afraid of anything else. I may not like it but I don't have to be afraid of it.

When I first started this journey, there were many times when the dark shadows of fear and discouragement loomed frighteningly over my thinking in the middle of the night. That's not so true anymore. Now, when I wake at 2:00am, which is not uncommon, I find it's a great time to talk with God. Those are some of the best times I've had.

◆

Memorizing scripture gives you the weapons you need to combat fear and discouragement. I encourage you to memorize these important verses:

- Isaiah 41:10
- Psalm 34:6
- Romans 12:12
- I Thessalonians 5:18

The enemy wants to keep us afraid but God has not given us a spirit of fear. He can fill you with the power, love and self-discipline to face your circumstances.

A Devastating Diagnosis

Our hopes were high as we went back to the Mayo Clinic on Friday, July 29th to meet with my pulmonologist. Just two days earlier, I'd been treated and cleared of brain cancer. Before that, the pulmonologist had given us hope that my lung cancer, the final remaining cancer, could be treated with a simple pill.

His somber expression quickly told us that wouldn't be the case. "John," he said, "I'm sorry to say that your cancer has spread. It's definitely stage four." He frowned and pursed his lips together as he paused. He glanced at Sharon before looking back at me. "It's not curable. But we can treat it."

I gripped Sharon's hand tighter and looked into her eyes, thankful to have her by my side through all of this.

"There are likely other cancer cells throughout your body that aren't visible to current technology. Chemotherapy and medication may delay the progression of the disease, but, eventually, the cancer will break through and grow again." He paused again to see how we were both handling the news. I swallowed hard and sat up a little straighter, never letting go of Sharon's hand. "The chemotherapy for this type of cancer will cause side effects that could make the treatment worse than the disease."

"And if I don't get the treatment?" I asked.

"I expect that you would have a few months to live."

"And if I have the chemo?"

"We can't say for sure. The survival rate is 20% to 40% after two years."

There was a long pause again. The air hung heavy with the news. Our hopes and prayers for an easy treatment had vanished in an instant. Sharon wiped a tear from her cheek.

The doctor continued. "John, at your stage of health, I readily admit that there is much we do not know and cannot predict. I'm sorry to say that, at this point, we are in the business of providing marginal benefits at the cost of some pretty bad side effects."

Sharon and I left in stunned silence. A nurse was kind enough to lead us to the scheduling desk to make my chemo appointment for the following week to start the next phase of my cancer treatment.

The flight back home to Fort Meyers seemed much longer than usual that night. Our conversation was not without hope, but far more somber than what was normal for us. After successfully battling COVID, mantel cell lymphoma, and then brain cancer, the thought of taking on yet another, even more grueling cancer treatment was daunting.

I woke up the next morning and looked out over a small body of water behind our house that I call Serenity Pond. Like my time beside the Root River in Lanesboro, Serenity Pond provides the perfect setting to watch the water and talk to my Heavenly Father. I breathed in the rich aroma of the flowering bushes planted along the shore and watched as a female wood duck paddled past me followed by five nearly grown ducklings. I prayed, remembering God's faithfulness and his many answers to prayer.

I also thought back over the last seven months. Our lives had been a blur of "chasing the cure" since January. The initial diagnosis came in and we jumped into months of chemo. Scans, function tests and MRI's revealed more cancer and, with God's help and the latest technology, it was treated and eliminated. But now this – a terminal diagnosis whichever way we looked at it. If I didn't get treatment, I'd be dead in a few months. If I do get treatment, I could still be dead in a few months.

I felt a strong need to take a time out from chasing the cure for a little while, to let the dust settle from everything the doctor told us, to pause and rest.

Later that day, Sharon and I went out for appetizers and drinks to spend some much needed time talking. The restaurant was on the twelfth floor of a hotel and our table sat on the balcony over-looking the water. The evening sun shimmered golden off the tops of the waves gently rocking the boats in the marina. Seagulls seemed to hang in the air, riding the steady coastal breeze. Tourists paused on the docks to take selfies as sailboats heading out for an evening cruise passed behind them. The beautiful view gave us a much needed higher perspective that coincided with our need for a higher perspective of my diagnosis. As we pondered and prayed, Sharon and I were reminded of other times in our 53 years of marriage when circumstances were bleak. Then God reminded us again of his faithfulness to provide the comfort and strength to get through.

This morning I awoke and went back out to my seat overlook-ing Serenity Pond. I felt a great sense that the burden of Friday's diagnosis had been lifted from my soul. The diagnosis didn't own me. I own it. And God owns me. I flung the backpack of that burden onto the Lord and I wasn't going to pick it up again. I've had a grin on my face ever since.

As for my treatments, we've decided to wait a little while and see how God leads. I'm leaning toward not getting them at all. My son summarized it so well in a letter to those praying for me, "I can go without the treatments and continue to feel great until the very end, when I'll feel bad for a little while. Or, I can take the treatments and feel bad all the time for a couple years – and then I still die." It's not an easy decision.

I want to honor and glorify God in my life and in the body he's given me. We all have a "best if used by" date on our earth suits. We just don't know when that date will come.

Jeremiah 29:11 (NIV) says, "For I know the plans I have for you, declares the Lord, plans to prosper you and not to harm you, plans to give you a hope and a future."

The question I keep asking myself is, *Wouldn't this plan also include heaven?*

How can you respond when there are setbacks in your situation?

Believe the promise of Jeremiah 29:11 (NIV). "For I know the plans I have for you, declares the Lord, plans to prosper you and not to harm you, plans to give you a future and a hope."

Is This God's Fault?

Did God cause this? It's a question that many people with serious health issues or in troubling situations might ask. We're all looking for THE reason why this is happening. Was it something I did? Was it because of a lifestyle choice? Was it something in my environment that is someone else's fault? Or, did God himself bring this on me?

Answer: I don't know, but I do know that he allowed it. My personal feeling is that he didn't cause my cancer or your personal health concern for that matter. Our fallen world is at fault and, ultimately, God will use it for his glory. It's a difficult thing to accept when it's our lives on the line, but our purpose as Christians, healthy or unhealthy, is to bring glory to the Father.

Does it really matter who caused it? If God is good, then he never does anything bad. Psalm 100:5 (NIV) says, "For the Lord is good and His love endures forever; His faithfulness continues through all generations." I think the question goes back to our own doubt and discouragement. Someone might say, *I'm not liking what God is doing right now and I'm finding reasons not to trust him anymore. If God caused this, I don't want to have anything to do with him.*

The truth is, this is life. Stuff happens. Good and bad. Solomon says in Ecclesiastes that there is a season for everything and God is in control of all of it. Sometimes, we may not like that idea because of what's going on, but God is still in control. We have to believe that.

God's perspective is this. Psalm 91:15 (NKJV) "He shall call upon me and I will answer him. I will be with him in trouble. I will deliver him and honor him." There are so many times in life when God doesn't necessarily save us from going through the trial, or the failure, or the sickness, but he promises to go through it with us. "He will never leave you nor forsake you." Deuteronomy 31:6 (NIV).

Personally, I've never questioned whether God caused my illness. But, if he caused it, he'll use it for his glory. If he didn't cause it, he'll use it for his glory.

I can rest in that.

◆

Acknowledge that God is good, even when your circumstances don't feel that way.

Focus on how God can use your challenges for his glory.

Difficult Decisions

I'm faced with difficult choices that I can't squirm out of. I have to choose between treatments that could potentially extend my life but are certain to cause severe side effects, or I can choose no treatments at all and accept my eventual fate.

How are we as Christians supposed to make decisions like that? Do we flip a coin? Proverbs 16:33 (TLB) says, "We toss the coin, but it is the Lord who controls its decision." I like flipping coins, but then, when I don't like the answer, I go for two out of three, or three out of five. We're also told to seek wise counsel, but I've been guilty of stacking the deck with people who agree with me. Some would say listen to your heart, but the Bible states that, "The heart is deceitful above all things, and desperately wicked; who can know it?" Jeremiah 17:19 (NKJV)

I think we can take great comfort in the knowledge that if we're already seeking God's will and prayerfully considering our circumstances, we're already in the stream. We're already moving in the flow of God's will. We have trusted him to guide us to this point and we can trust that he will continue. We can confidently make a decision knowing that God will direct us.

I like Hannah Whitall Smith's book, The Christian's Secret to a Happy Life, originally published in 1875. She lays out four ways that God reveals his will to his followers.

Scripture – What does the Bible say about what you are facing?

Circumstances – He leads, you follow. He opens doors.

Common Sense – God gave it to you. He is a God of order, not disorder.

Holy Spirit Impressions – Is God nudging you in a certain direction?

God's voice will always be in harmony with itself, no matter how many ways he speaks. In the end, there should be a divine sense of "oughtness" about our decision.

At the start of my journey, I made the decision to take chemo for the mantel cell lymphoma. That proved to be the right decision and we were successful. Then I was diagnosed with brain cancer. I went through the decision-making process a little quicker, accepting that treatment as well. Now, with my current diagnosis and the threat of difficult treatments, I have another chance to waffle a bit.

I had to ask myself, *What's the last thing God told you to do when all this started? Get the chemo.* So that's what I'm going to do.

Psalm 139:23,24 (NIV) says, "Search me, God, and know my heart; test me and know my anxious thoughts. See if there is any offensive way in me, and *lead me in the way everlasting*" (italics mine). We can ask God. Have faith in him. Pray and believe that he'll lead us in our decisions. "For it is God who works in you to will and to act in order to fulfill His good purpose." (Philippians 2:13 NIV)

I trust that God is driving. I'll make a decision and then adjust if he steers in a different direction. "Being confident of this, that He who began a good work in you will carry it on to completion until the day of Christ Jesus." (Philippians 1:6 NIV)

◆

If you are struggling with a decision, what is the last thing God instructed you to do?

God's leading may come from scripture, circumstances, common sense and an impression from the Holy Spirit.

You can rest in the promise that "He who began a good work in you will carry it on to completion until the day of Jesus Christ." Philippians 1:6

Continuing the Fight

The idea of going through chemo and willingly inflicting pain and suffering on myself in the hope of a 20% chance that I might extend my life an additional two years is not a pleasant thought. But to quote my friend who encouraged me to go through chemo the first time, "John, this is not about you. You have a sphere of influence. You have people watching you. Your job is to take the treatment, do your part, and trust God for the rest. The results are up to God. You don't get to pick the time. You just have to keep on trucking."

The truth is that I did have people in my life asking me not to give up yet. They wanted me to do what I could do for as long as I could do it. If the chemo got to be too bad, I could always stop. I also wanted to see the results of a new chest scan and brain MRI scheduled for October 10th.

I was still vacillating on getting the chemo when I went to my

Tuesday morning Bible Study. The section of scripture we were studying was the last portion of Philippians 4. There's a lot of great messages in that chapter. Don't be anxious about anything. Pray about everything. The peace of God will guard your hearts and minds. They're all very familiar verses, but the Holy Spirit pulled something else out for my attention, verses 21 and 22 (NIV). "Greet all God's people in Christ Jesus. The brothers and sisters who are with me send greetings. All God's people here send you greetings, *especially those who belong to Caesar's household*" (italics mine).

It's so amazing how the Holy Spirit uses scripture. What we would normally consider "throw away" verses, the Holy Spirit instead spoke to me and said, *Paul was a prisoner at the very highest ranks of the Roman Empire, and there were members of Caesar's household who became believers because of Paul's influence. They became part of the Bride of Christ because Paul was in a difficult spot.* The Holy Spirit seemed to say to me, *That's kind of where you're at, John. You're in a difficult spot, but you're still talking to people and it's making a difference.*

That verse encouraged me to stay the course and keep doing what I was doing. Every one of us is in a place where God is speaking to us, and also through us. I needed to stay available. I still had life. I still had options. There were still things to do. God was with me. I wanted to see what was going to happen.

On August 31st I drove to Tampa for my first big boy chemo treatment. Surprisingly, it was a great day. After blood tests, doctor appointments, a delicious lunch, followed by three hours of infusions, I was back home in bed by 10 o'clock and slept great. Even the next morning, I felt no ill effects from the chemo. I was reveling in God's marvelous orchestration of my day.

Then the hammer fell. I was beaten down. The previous infusions I had for mantel cell lymphoma felt like the Fisher-Price kiddie version of chemo. This one was like WWE Smackdown wrestling. My teeth hurt, my tongue, my heart, my joints, everything felt like it was getting whacked.

I suddenly had a new appreciation for Job. He lost everything, suffering extreme physical affliction, all while maintaining the perspective of God's sovereignty over his circumstances. My discomfort became the object of my full attention. My capacity to think or feel any perspective beyond the pain was almost gone. I really didn't care about the big picture. I only cared about me.

I leaned on the promise of Philippians 4:13 (NKJV) when Paul says, "I can do all things through Christ who strengthens me." I like to meditate on it in the Amplified Bible Classic Edition. "I have strength for all things in Christ Who empowers me. [I am ready for anything and equal to anything through Him Who infuses inner strength into me; I am self-sufficient in Christ's sufficiency]."

I am self-sufficient in Christ's sufficiency. Of course, this doesn't mean that we are self-reliant, standing on our own strength and ability to face the challenge. No, it's only through our total dependence on him and his provision that we can stand. Then the Holy Spirit infuses us with his inner strength to do what God would have us do.

Philippians 4:19 (NKJV) goes on to say, "And my God shall supply all your need according to His riches in glory by Christ Jesus."

My daily prayer has become, *Lord, help me to think correctly about this situation.* And he reminds me of Psalm 27:14 (NKJV). "Wait on the Lord; Be of good courage and He shall strengthen your heart; wait, I say, on the Lord."

So that's what I'm going to do.

◆

God speaks to us and through us. God can use you in your present circumstances to reach and encourage others.

Are you still "on assignment" for God?

We are sufficient in Christ's sufficiency. We can be ready for anything because he infuses us with inner strength and peace. How have you experienced his sufficiency in your journey?

Is There Still Hope for Healing?

There was finally some good news. I was back in my neurologist's office October 13th, two days after a brain MRI and chest CT scan. The doctor turned the computer screen toward me as he pulled up my file.

"Here's your brain MRI from July," he said, taking his pen and pointing out two small dots on the image. "You can clearly see the lesions that we were concerned about." He pushed a button on the keyboard and a new image appeared. "Now, here's your latest MRI from last Monday." He turned from the monitor, raised his eyebrows and smiled. "The scan is clear." He pointed back to the areas where the cancer had been. "There's nothing there. The Gamma Knife surgery was successful. The cancer is gone. Congratulations." There were no other treatments or testing to be done. My brain cancer was gone. It could not have been better news.

I hoped for an equally good report about my lung cancer from my thoracic doctor. If the scans revealed that the tumor had shrunk, then the chemo infusions were working and our plan would be set going forward. I connected with the doctor on Zoom later that day and, in similar fashion, he pulled up my original CT scan of my chest with the tumor visible in my right lung.

"I'm sure this looks all too familiar," he said. "This is your scan from July, The tumor really hadn't grown much since it was first discovered when you were in the hospital with COVID." The scan was replaced with a full screen shot of the doctor. He seemed to sigh and his expression softened before he spoke again. "John, I'm sorry to say that's no longer true."

A new image filled the screen. A black and white cross section of my chest appeared. In CT scans, lung tissue appears black. Denser tissue like bone, muscle and tumors, appear white. In the center of my right lung was a large white spot and it was much bigger than in the previous image.

"The tumor has doubled in size and it's growing quickly," said the doctor. "Obviously, the present chemo isn't working. I'd like to propose an alternative."

I was stunned. After my morning appointment with the neurologist, I was expecting good news. It took a couple seconds for me to respond. "What would happen if we stopped the chemo all together?"

The doctor shifted in his chair. "I would estimate that you'd be on oxygen by Christmas, maybe two or three months. But, if the new chemo is effective," he tried to sound encouraging, "you could have a year or more."

In an instant, I was back to a terminal diagnosis.

Looking to My Future

I have two pictures in my office. One is a photo of me up at Lake of the Woods holding a big walleye. Good memories. The other is a picture of Jesus with his arms draped over a man who looks a little like me. It speaks to me about the compassion of Jesus, especially during this time. "John, my son, you're not going to figure it all out, but I'm with you. I'm with you."

I go into my future trusting that Jesus still has his arms wrapped around me. I don't know what the coming months will bring, but I do know that "the Lord is good" (Psalm 100:5 NKJV). "His mercy is everlasting, and His truth endures to all generations." I will continue to ask, seek and knock for healing because the Bible invites us to do that. I will also take the next round of chemo for the sake of my wife and family. But I will trust God with the results.

A pastor friend of mine had a sign hanging in his office that read, "Faith which refuses to face indisputable facts is but little faith." I've thought about that a lot. There are indisputable facts about my situation. The tests say what they say. Facts are facts. Unless God steps in, I'm like Elisha: I'm sick with the illness from which I'm going to die. Trying to buy more time so that God can work a miracle doesn't seem to make much sense. The God who can heal me is the same God who could have prevented this disease. We're at a place in my care where we're just trying to extend the expiration date.

But I am at peace. I have spent a lifetime in God's Word and I know that there's so much more to God's plan than what's going on here. The whole point of all of this is to glorify God. It's not about me. It's not about my survival. It's about honoring God. I will stay on assignment. I will continue to talk to people about our loving, compassionate Father. And I will be grateful for all of God's wonderful blessings – whatever my future holds.

Philippians 1: 18-21 (NIV) "Yes, and I will continue to rejoice, for I know that through your prayers and God's provision of the Spirit of Jesus Christ what has happened to me will turn out for my deliverance. I eagerly expect and hope that I will in no way be ashamed, but will have sufficient courage so that now as always Christ will be exalted in my body, whether by life or by death. For to me, to live is Christ and to die is gain."

My hope and prayer is that you will come to that place of desiring to honor God in all areas of your life. If you are healthy, thank God, and live the rest of your life for him. Finish well. If you are battling disease, fight hard, use whatever tools are at your disposal, but trust God to guide, to comfort, and to heal according to his will. He is with you every step of the way and in all circumstances.

Scripture

Chapter 3
Proverbs 3:5,6
I Thessalonians 5:18
1 Peter 5:7
Matthew 11:28-30

Chapter 4
Proverbs 3:5,6
Psalm 118:17
Exodus 23:25,26
1 Peter 2:24

Chapter 7
Hebrews 13:5b
Matthew 7:7-11
Psalm 18:30
2 Kings 13:14
Proverbs 3:5,6
James 1:2,3
Psalm 100:5
2 Corinthians 12:9
Deut. 31:6
Isaiah 41:10
Hebrews 13:6
Psalm 18:6
Psalm 31:15
Psalm 115:3
Jeremiah 29:11
Psalm 20:7
Zechariah 4:6b
Psalm 139:16

Chapter 7 (cont)
Psalm 115:3
Jeremiah 29:11
Psalm 20:7
Zechariah 4:6b
Psalm 139:16

Chapter 9
Psalm 27:13,14
Romans 15:13
Psalm 103:2-4

Chapter 10
Psalm 103
Isaiah 41:10
Psalm 27:13,14

Chapter 13
James 1:2
Isaiah 41:10
Luke 12:27,28

Chapter 14
Psalm 18:29
Chapter 15
Ephesians 2:6,7

Scripture

Chapter 17
1 Thessalonians 5:18
Psalm 23:4
Psalm 91:15
Kings 2:2
Psalm 31:15
Psalm 18:30
Psalm 115:3
Hebrews 13:6
Deuteronomy 31:6
Romans 8:28
Hebrews 13:8
Psalm 103:2-4
Psalm 30:9
Psalm 34:2
James 1:2

Chapter 19
James 5:14,15
Philippians 4:13
Mark 11:22-24
Matthew 26:39

Chapter 20
Isaiah 41:10
2 Timothy 1:7
Psalm 34:6
1 Peter 5:7
Philippians 4:8

Chapter 20 (cont)
2 Corinthians 10:5
Colossians 3:2
Romans 12:2
Romans 12:12

Chapter 21
Jeremiah 29:11

Chapter 22
Psalm 100:5
Psalm 91:15
Deuteronomy 31:6

Chapter 23
Proverbs 16:33
Jeremiah 17:19
Psalm 139:23,24
Philippians 2:13
Philippians 1:6

Chapter 24
Philippians 4:21,22
Philippians 4:13
Philippians 4:19
Psalm 27:14
Chapter 26
Psalm 100:5
Philippians 1:18-21